Keep Your College Daughter Safe:

161 Ways College Women Can Prevent Sexual Assault

Richard Hart

Verum Publishing and Verum Press
Atlanta, Georgia

ISBN: 0-9787476-3-1
2nd 9 780978 747633

Verum Publishing (and Verum Press)
10383 Tara Blvd # 257
Jonesboro GA 30236
www.VerumPress.com

My thanks to God for giving me the
inspiration and ability to make a difference.

And to my mother for having raised me to
respect all people and to bring me an awareness
that we're all in this together.
And for being a great mom.

Thanks also to Apex Book Awards for
recognizing *Keep Your Daughter Safe* as a book
that will make a difference. Winner writing
excellence; Grand Award Winner 2008.

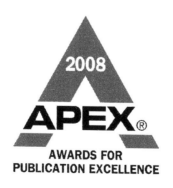

This book was written by a man – a man who was raised to respect and appreciate women for the incredible human beings they are.

> **More than half of all women in the United States will experience physical or sexual assault at some point during their lifetimes.** Source: United States Department of Justice

NOTHING GIVES A MAN THE RIGHT
TO LAY HIS HANDS UPON
A WOMAN OR A CHILD.

The goal of this book is to educate women about the situations that may lead to sexual assault and to help them avoid or deal with those situations.

The suggestions found inside are the culmination of my experience pursuing a degree in Criminal Science, additional crime prevention training I received through my work with Aid to Victims and Witnesses and law enforcement agencies, targeted readings on crime and crime prevention, and finally, from the countless stories I've been told by women who've suffered at the hands of predatory men.

Much of this writing mirrors public lectures I have given on victim-avoidance strategies.

If just one woman benefits from this information, my job is complete. However, my hope is that the statistics outlined in Chapter One will fall due to increased awareness affected by suggestions found in this book.

No woman asks to be raped, any more than somebody driving a nice car asks to have it stolen. BUT, be very clear – if half of all cars were being stolen, Americans would demand action, and things would change. For some reason, it seems to be acceptable in the United States that one out of every two women is the victim of sexual or physical abuse.

THIS MUST END!

Most men do not understand that many women view half of the population as potential predators.

Think about this: If a man is robbed, he hands over his wallet, money clip, or credit cards, and the bad guy leaves. Even under the worst circumstances, men generally have no need to fear an event known as sexual assault. On the other hand, if a woman is held up for her car or purse, the chance of her becoming the victim of a sexual assault is also present.

This threat does not hang over the heads of most men, so it is difficult for men to relate to or understand why so many women view all men as potential predators. The societal implications of this perception are huge.

This book is divided into two primary sections. The first section, Chapters 1 through 5, describe the emotional, physical and economic impacts on victims and society, myth versus reality of rape and sexual assault, distinctions pertaining to the definitions of assaults, how assaults happen, etc. The second section, Chapters 6 through 13, discusses situational methods any woman can use to reduce her odds of becoming yet one more statistic on a list that is already way too long. Chapter 14 covers methods of thwarting an actual attack.

It is time for things to change.

I hope this book makes a difference in your life and in the lives of women across America.

Richard Hart

Compact Discs of this book are available.

**A © Copyrighted Scenario DVD
has also been produced.
Please visit the website listed below to
view or hear clips of the DVD or CD.**

**The website also has SPECIAL OFFERS
on multiple book purchases and bulk discounts
as well as information on
arranging public presentations.**

www.AWorldWithoutRape.org

Table of Contents

IF YOU DO NOT LIKE TO READ, please
GO STRAIGHT TO CHAPTERS 6 - 15.

Chapter One

Statistics

IF YOU DO NOT LIKE TO READ,
please go straight to chapters 6 - 15.

FACT: More than **half of all women** will experience a sexual or physical assault at some point in their lifetimes.[i]

Whenever I repeat this statistic to a woman, any woman, she reflects on the women she knows now or from her past, and then informs me that the number is **low**.

This statistic is gathered from reports to crisis centers, women's shelters, and other victim support groups who aid women caught in these situations. The numbers from these groups indicate that the FBI statistics listed in its Uniform Crime Report are inordinately low. Women's beliefs that reporting these incidents will bring about further embarrassment, traumatic reliving of the attack, perceived hassle and continued disregard for women, could all be potential factors for low reporting rates.

FACT: As many as 1 in 5 women will be sexually assaulted during their lifetimes.[ii]

The reason this number appears to be at odds with the first statistic is due to the fact that a) the first statistic quotes sexual *and* physical assaults; and b) this FBI statistic is the result of crime data compilations stated in the Uniform Crime Report. Even the FBI acknowledges that the rapes reported, and therefore counted in its crime statistics, represent only between 5 and 10 percent of all actual rapes taking place in America. Further, the Uniform Crime Report only counts completed rapes; it does not address the issues of non-rape sexual assaults or uncompleted rapes (attempted rape). In their 1992 report, *Rape in America: A Report to the Nation* – the National Victim Center reported that 9 out of 10 rapes go unreported.[iii] The Bureau of Justice Statistics reports: "Fewer than 5% of attempted rapes or completed rapes were reported to law enforcement officials [in the college environment.]" This means a mere 1 out of 20 rapes is reported in the college environment.

IF only 1 in 10 rapes is reported,

AND since the FBI's Uniform Crime Report numbers show that in 2004 (the most recent year for which statistics are available) there were 94,635 reported rapes of females over the age of 12 (rapes of girls younger than 12 constitute child abuse and are not counted in the Uniform Crime Report as "rapes"),

THEN we can extrapolate and conclude that approximately 946,000 actual rapes took place in the United States in 2004. (These numbers do not regard non-rape sexual assaults, which catapult the victim numbers into the stratosphere.)

Based upon this information, a woman is raped approximately every 35 seconds in America.

FACT: 1 in 4 college women will be sexually assaulted during her tenure as a student.[iv] This too, is a Department of Justice statistic.

Think of yourself and 3 of your friends. It is a statistical probability that **one of you will be sexually assaulted during your college years.**

FACT: 4 out of 5 women who are raped *personally know* the perpetrator.[v]

This means that 80% of all rape victims know the person who rapes them! We will address this topic in greater detail later. For the time being, you must understand that the rape events we hear about in the media are almost always "glamour stories" used to sell newspapers or advertising time for television news. But those events only represent about 20% of all sexual assaults.

THESE STATISTICS ARE REPULSIVE. They are indicative of a society that has become so complacent that it (society) deems the abuse of women to be inevitable or even acceptable. Media, lawyers and other quasi-public entities have successfully shifted the blame for rapes and other sexual assaults to the women who suffer these attacks.

Consider this: A man withdraws money from an ATM, and is robbed, at which point, the police, his wife, his friends, and the owner of the ATM all say, "You should have been more careful. By withdrawing that money in public, you were *just asking to be robbed.*" Yeah, right! I don't think so. **He did not ask to be robbed, any more than any woman ever asks to be raped.**

Please know: this book is not about becoming paranoid, but about becoming aware.

Chapter Two

The Vast Repercussions of Sexual Assault

There have been numerous books and literally thousands of articles dealing with the mental, physical, and economic effects experienced by victims of sexual assault.

For instance, students who have been acquaintance raped by someone at school may drop out. Workers, who have been attacked by someone at the office, may quit the company, file lawsuits, or both. Women experiencing severe, although completely normal, mental responses to an attack, may watch their families fall apart due to family members' inability to effectively deal with the aftermath of an assault.

The results from one study that surveyed 3,000 women across 32 campuses found that 31% of women identified as rape victims had contemplated suicide at some point after the attack.[vi] This rate is 13 times higher than women who have not been victimized by rape.

It is impossible to know just how deep the true impact of rape and sexual assault runs. There is no way of telling how many divorces, school dropouts, sick days, employment terminations, reductions in grade point averages, or other seemingly "everyday" events have been impacted by the responses or reactions to sexual assaults.

The economic costs are equally staggering. With estimated costs between 110 and 127 BILLION DOLLARS per year, sexual assaults experience the highest per-victim costs of all crimes. These figures do not include child sexual abuse or the impact on law enforcement budgets.

In comparison, the victim costs associated with robbery is a mere $4 billion. At what point do we arrive at a place where we as a society say, "Enough!"?

The purpose of this chapter is not to minimize the reactions experienced by victims of rape and sexual assault; nor is it an attempt to deal with these responses. Rather, the goal is to explore the wide range of responses and to affirm that no matter what a woman's response, it should NOT be considered an abnormal reaction to the traumatic event of rape or sexual assault.

A STUDY OF RAPE VICTIMS

In his study titled *The Mental Health Impact of Rape*, Dean Kilpatrick, Ph.D., found the following:

- Almost one-third of rape victims experienced post-traumatic stress disorder.

- Rape victims were 3 times more likely than women who were not victims of a violent crime to experience a major depressive episode.

- A victim of rape was 13 times more likely than a non-crime victim to have attempted suicide.

- 1 in 8 rape victims has attempted suicide.

- Rape victims were 13 times more likely to have a problem with alcohol.

- Rape victims were 26 times more likely to have some type of drug abuse problem.

A myriad of other studies through the years report similar findings.

Because the fallout from sexual abuse in our country is real, and extraordinarily vast, it is incumbent upon us to recognize some of the signs that indicate a rape or sexual assault has taken place.

In a poll of women who had been raped, more than 70% did not want their families to know they had been sexually violated. And, we must not forget, these numbers reflect only reported attacks. Statistics indicate that approximately 1 in 10 rapes or sexual assaults are actually reported to the authorities. In a Department of Justice report, the writing cited that **a mere 1 in 20 rapes is reported in the college environment.**

Whether the attacks are reported or not, virtually every victim experiences severe reactions associated with the trauma created by a sexual assault.

A WOMAN'S MENTAL STATE DURING, AND IMMEDIATELY FOLLOWING, AN ATTACK

Obviously, different women respond differently. The media has successfully sold the public on the portrayal of the "hysterical victim," to such an extent that if a woman is not hysterical after being raped; we (the public) are of the mindset that no attack must have really taken place. It has taken 30 years for it to finally be understood that a woman is just as likely to engage in "complete withdrawal" after a sexual assault, as she is to be the hysterical victim.

During the actual attack, many women will "freeze" from fright, or from their body's attempt to disassociate from the attack. It is not unusual for this "paralysis" to spill over into the post-attack period, where a woman may report the events of the attack to authorities almost as if she had

7

viewed the attack through a window, as opposed to having personally experienced the assault.

Psychological disorganization (the appearance of being disoriented) and a form of stress-induced amnesia known as psychogenic amnesia are both also normal responses experienced by women in the aftermath of a sexual attack.

Picture yourself lost in a crowded, downtown section of a major city at night. If someone (even someone you knew) were to approach you to ask for directions, you might at first, hesitate with a distinct sense of "not getting it" or failing to understand their question. This is similar to a psychological disorganization or a disoriented reaction.

Now picture yourself lost in the same downtown area, but then being asked three hours later about a car crash that had occurred across the street from where you were standing while you were lost. It could be difficult to remember the specific details of the accident. This is a loose example of psychogenic amnesia. This sense of "trying to find your way" or intense feeling of being lost, is similar to the sensation experienced by some victims of a sexual assault, thus creating a case where certain components of the memory of the actual attack may be blotted out.

During a sexual assault, a victim could be experiencing a very real fear of death, a dream-state equivalent of "this can't be happening" or a drug- or alcohol-induced inability to even know what is taking place. In any of these scenarios, it might be difficult for a woman to remember much about the attack or the attacker(s), unless it happened to be a situation where she knew the attacker beforehand (date rape for example).

LONG-TERM AFTER-EFFECTS

Sexual assaults are so physically invasive and mentally disruptive that in the weeks, months, or even years following an attack a woman could experience episodes of depression, anger, unexplainable mood swings, feelings of guilt, or self-doubt, isolation, or a sense of loss of control. The inconsistency of these thoughts, feelings, or emotional states, could place any victim on an emotional roller-coaster.

Sleep Disorders

Sleep might be continually disrupted by the trauma and the semi-conscious "reliving" of the attack, prohibiting a woman from getting a sound night's rest. Conversely, a woman could find herself sleeping excessively, which would indicate more of a depressive response.

Flashbacks Associated With the Attack

Some women have reported statements such as: "Every time I see a guy in long shorts with no shirt, I re-experience the attack" or "The memories feel so real, it's like I'm there all over again." These feelings of reliving the attack can be especially pervasive if the victim has not told anyone about the attack and/or the perpetrator is a family member or someone the woman sees on a regular basis.

Depression

Depression is one of the most common responses to a sexual assault. It can result from self-blame for the occurrence of the incident or from the invasive nature of the attack itself.

Symptoms of depression could take the form of excessive sleep patterns, severe weight gain or loss, drug or alcohol abuse, suicidal thoughts or attempts at suicide, or destructive/high risk behaviors (behaviors which could be likened to suicidal patterns, but that create circumstances where if death did occur, it would not be labeled a suicide).

Fear and Paranoia

Some women experience intense, even unrealistic, fears which cause them to begin jumping at the slightest sound, viewing all men as potential predators, repeating panic-inducing thoughts such as, "What if it happens again?" or "I can't let this happen again." These victims begin to maintain a manic state of hyper-vigilance, where anything and everything taking place in their environment enters their consciousness. Little things a woman may never have noticed now attract her full attention. This further decreases a victim's energy levels and overall effectiveness in life.

Feelings of Powerlessness or Loss of Control

A significant aspect of any sexual assault is the perpetrator's demonstrating total control over his victim. This is a significant part of the attacker's "payoff." In response to having been so thoroughly dominated in the rape situation, many women are left with a sense of no control. A woman may now feel she needs to control even the smallest details of her life in order to compensate for the total lack of control she felt during the attack. However, since no person can control every detail of their life, situations will arise when a woman who has been raped will feel completely helpless. This woman will not know what has triggered this feeling, yet it can likely be traced directly back to the attack.

One woman's story went like this: "I was driving down the freeway, when all-of-a-sudden, I had this horrible feeling of dread come over me. 'What if another driver didn't stay on his side of the road?' I became so traumatized with the possibility of this occurring that I had to pull over and have a friend pick me up."

Severe Mood Swings

A woman may appear to have recovered from an attack; however, she may be happy one moment, and crying a few minutes later due to a reminder of the attack dredged-up by her subconscious. The trigger could be something as simple as someone pouring her a glass of water, which the victim may have linked in her mind to being the way she was served a drugged drink which led to a rape.

A woman may also experience extreme anger over a trivial incident – one that people who have not been victims of sexual assault would view and label as "no-big-deal."

Withdrawal and Avoidance

Withdrawal and Avoidance are two very common responses to sexual assaults.

Withdrawal could mean complete and total isolation from other people. It could be physical withdrawal from a specific environment, such as a young woman who decides to leave college or move out of her apartment complex, due to constant reminders of the attack represented by these locations. The withdrawal could be from a partner or family member who did not respond in a sympathetic manner to news of the attack, or who, because they did not know how to respond, offered, from the victim's perspective, an "inappropriate" response.

Some women gain weight or wear two or three extra layers of clothing in an attempt to "cover-up" or "withdraw." Part of the psychology behind these actions is the belief that by making herself "less attractive," she can prevent a repeat attack. An additional negative related to this situation is the fact that the victim has now also associated (or placed) part of the blame for the attack on her own appearance or actions.

Avoidance may seem similar to withdrawal, but there are substantive differences. The withdrawal is really pulling away from anything and everything that could in any way be associated with the attack. A woman could pull away from relationships with all men or leave a college, city, or job behind. The scale of withdrawal behavior is much larger than avoidance. In avoidance, the woman will decide to no longer walk past the building where the rape took place. She may not go back to the bar where she met the man who took her to his place and attacked her. Her goal is to rid herself of reminders of the event, similar to someone who changes a radio station when a song is played that brings back an unpleasant memory.

WHAT CAN YOU DO IF SOMEONE YOU KNOW IS RAPED?

As stated earlier, these mental states are all standard reactions to an attack. There is no specific timeframe for recovery, since different victims respond differently and since many attacks may bear components beyond the actual sexual assault, such as the use of violence or drugs, which may evoke additional negative responses from the victim.

It is extremely difficult to get through the aftermath of a sexual assault without some type of assistance. Help could come from a friend or family member, a psychiatrist, a member of the clergy, a support group, etc. The important thing to know is in almost all cases help must come from somewhere.

If you notice one or more of these behaviors occurring with a friend, where the moods or mental states are a complete reversal of that friend's normal behavior patterns, there is a possibility that an attack may have taken place. Tell your friend you have noticed a change in her behavior and that if she wishes to talk about the situation, you will hold everything she tells you in strictest confidence. **(IMPORTANT: If you make this promise, you must keep this promise!** There is nothing worse than reluctantly agreeing to trust a friend or family member only to find that trust has been breached.)

If a friend or family member has approached you with the information that she has suffered a rape or sexual assault, the most important thing to remember is that your friend did not bring this upon herself. By confiding in you, your friend is attempting to make sense of the event and may also be attempting to regain part of the control she feels she's lost.

As her friend, you must try to assist her in regaining a sense of trust and certainty. If you do not feel capable of adequately dealing with the situation, try to convince your friend to speak with a counselor or go to a crisis center that specializes in dealing with victims of sexual assault. You can also offer to accompany her to the meeting(s) as a sign of ongoing friendship and support.

If you are a victim of sexual assault, you should NOT try to deal with this on your own. You should seek outside help. Please review the *Resources* Section at the end of this book

Chapter Three

Myth versus Reality

MYTH: Rapists and sexual predators are easy to spot; they fit a specific profile.

REALITY: First, 4 out of 5 assault victims know their assailant. That's 80%! If the perpetrators readily fit into an easy-to-recognize profile, far fewer attacks would occur.

Second, one of the highest-profile cases of date rape in recent years occurred in 2003. The case involved one of the heirs to a major cosmetics company fortune; a man named Andrew Luster. This man was a good-looking guy. He would meet women in bars, take them back to his place, drug them and rape them. He jumped his $10 million bail during his trial, but was convicted in absentia on multiple counts of rape, poisoning, and drug possession. He was given a sentence of 124 years. More importantly, this was a good-looking man whom most women would never have suspected of engaging in these practices.

MYTH: Women say "no" just because they've been raised or conditioned to do so. Women enjoy sex just as much as men. Therefore "no" doesn't really mean "no."

REALITY: It is immaterial whether women enjoy sex less or even more than men. Every woman has the right to decide where, when, and with whom she will engage in sexual activity. When a woman exercises her right to say "no," it is within her rights to say "no" and to expect a man to honor that statement.

MYTH: Women who drink with the guys or dress provocatively are "asking for it."

REALITY: There is no law forbidding women to consume alcohol and, with the exception of public nudity, there is no law stating how women must dress. I have never met a victim of sexual assault who acted as though she wanted to be raped. This attitude is insulting, and it is unconscionable that in the 21st century, we would still treat such a heinous crime in this manner. If we follow this line of thinking to its logical conclusion, then a store owner who doesn't place inventory control tags on his merchandise must want people to steal from him, right?? Wrong!

HOWEVER, we cannot ignore the huge role alcohol plays in many assault situations. Not because of its impact on women, but because of its influence on men. A physically aggressive man who has been drinking becomes more likely to get into a fight and a belligerent man becomes more belligerent. Alcohol often serves as a catalyst to move men into behavior patterns they would never consider if they were sober. Put some alcohol in him, and all-of-a-sudden, an otherwise apparently respectful man (who is not getting his way sexually) is no longer able or willing to hear the word, "No."

MYTH: If I steer clear of men of a particular race or ethnicity, I will be safe.

REALITY: If 80% of all sexual assaults occur in situations where the victim knows her assailant, and if we assume that most people generally date within their race, we can safely conclude the race card plays a very small role in sexual attacks. The fact that race is so frequently brought up during high profile rape cases is simply another attempt to blame women, to keep the races divided, and to deflect attention from the real problem: that the sexual assault of women is a tolerated practice in America. There is a 70% likelihood that a white rapist will rape a white victim and that a black rapist will rape a black victim.[vii]

MYTH: Rape is a spontaneous act committed by sex-starved or crazed deviants.

REALITY: Most rapes are committed by men who have consumed too much alcohol or who have carefully planned the attack. Sexual predators usually stake their victims. They may live in the same apartment complex or work in the same office building and have positioned themselves to know the comings and goings of their victims. They then wait for the right opportunity to strike.

Make no mistake, spontaneous and aggressive sexual assaults do occur, but with much less frequency than we are led to believe by the media.

MYTH: Carrying a weapon or taking self-defense classes will protect me.

REALITY: If a woman has to rely on self-defense, it's already too late. In all but a few situations, self-defense techniques are useless. Weapons can also give women a false sense of security causing them to place themselves in environments or situations they would never enter had they not been in possession of a weapon.

First, about self-defense. The average adult male weighs approximately 175 pounds. The average adult female weighs approximately 130 pounds. This means that, on average, men outweigh women by 45 pounds.

Since women generally do not grow up with physical fighting as a natural tendency, few women realize that if you take two extremely skilled boxers, and one of the two is 20 pounds lighter than the other, the fighter weighing less will lose to his heavier opponent almost every time. A woman stands **virtually no chance** physically against a man outweighing her by 45 pounds.

While self-defense lessons are not altogether a bad idea, a woman schooled in self-defense may develop a false sense of security. She may feel that she can handle any situation which may arise and, unfortunately, all-too-often this is not the case. Add alcohol to this equation, and all bets are off.

On the subject of weapons: There are 2 types of weapons: close-quarter and long-range. Without getting into a lot of detail, a long-range weapon would be a gun or a propellant such as pepper spray. Knives, sticks, keys, or other hand-held items of combat are close-quarter (close-range) weapons. Very few women carry guns. And of those who do, having a gun won't do much good if it's in the trunk of a car or buried at the bottom of a purse. The same goes for pepper spray. Close-quarter weapons are completely useless unless you can use them to take an attacker by surprise.

Example of a close-quarter surprise: A woman has her house key in her hand when she is attacked; her attacker doesn't see the key, and during the struggle, the victim gouges her attacker in his eye with her key. This would constitute a surprise response to an attack with a close-quarter weapon.

In sexual assault situations, weapons can easily be taken and used on the victim; the best defense is always remaining acutely aware of your surroundings and attempting to avoid environments or situations which could lead to, or result in, an attack.

As we can see, the common misperceptions of perpetrators of rape, will oftentimes lead women into a false sense of security. Women must remain aware of their surroundings at all times, not just when they are in a "bad part of town" or on a blind date.

Purchase additional copies for
your friends' daughters.

Purchase additional copies for
your nieces.

Purchase additional copies for
your neighbors' daughters.

Go to www.**VerumPress**.com

Together, we can end rape in America.

Chapter Four

Attacker Profiles and Their Methods of Operation

There are two types of sexual assailants: *Serial* and *Situational*.

The Serial Assailant

The Serial Assailant is also known as a "predator." He knows the law, and he does not care about it. He often chooses his victims very carefully. He will leave his residence intent on finding a victim. These are the "big story" guys – criminals with 5, 10, or even 20 assaults to their credit.

The Serial Assailant is easier to combat than his Situational Assailant counterpart. The predator's goal is to either: abduct and remove his victim to a quiet location or attack the victim in her own home. The reason this assailant is easier to combat or fend off, is that the predator is very similar to a burglar; his mission is to accomplish his goal quickly, easily, and with unnoticed movement. Anything that disrupts one of these 3 patterns will generally disrupt his attack plan causing him to seek an alternate victim.

Studies have shown the predator is less likely to attack a woman who moves with certainty and purpose as she walks. He is less likely to attempt entry into a home with a dog or where he feels a second person might also reside. He is less likely to force entry into a home when he knows, that on a hot summer night, a home with an open sliding glass door is likely only one or two doors away.

The predator may use drugs to render his victims unable to stop an attack. This Serial Assailant, again, has already carefully planned his attack. He is already carrying the drug vial in his pocket. He has already chosen which bar he will frequent. He is already looking for the woman sitting alone, while her friends are out on the dance floor. He may even have already picked out his target victim, before he even gets to the bar. There is nothing about his movement or agenda that is anything other than purposeful. The only thing rendering him *situational* would be *failing*. Any man who carries a date-rape drug with him is a Sexual Predator; not a Situational Assailant.

The predator relies upon the fact that his victims are distracted or are engaged in what might be considered careless behaviors (for example, leaving doors or windows open or unlocked, leaving drinks unattended while using the restroom, etc.). The Serial Assailant's movements are stealth in nature. For his intended victim to remain aware and/or exercise caution will oftentimes thwart his plans.

The Situational Assailant

The Situational Assailant fits no specific criminal profile. He may be married with children, single, a church-goer, a good guy to his neighbors, and so on. Additionally, his methods and psychology change or vary depending on circumstances. Between his lack of a specific profile and the methodology behind his attack patterns, the situational assailant is much more difficult to deal with or stop than his predator counterpart.

For example, the Situational Assailant might be driving to the store, see and pick up a hitchhiker, and then spontaneously assault her. Or, he could be walking down a street, see a cute 16-year-old and, in the absence of other people, drag her into the bushes and rape her. This type of attacker can be easily influenced by external stimuli such as alcohol, drugs, or even something as simple as watching a suggestive movie.

The most difficult *situational assailant* to deal with is the Date Rapist. While still falling into the *situational assailant* category, this is a man who has not intentionally walked into a bar, attended a party, or entered a woman's home after a date, with the intent of assaulting her.

Here are a few examples that demonstrate how a Date Rapist operates or how a date rape may occur.

Example 1: One of your friends sets you up with one of her co-workers. He picks you up and takes you to dinner. He is the "perfect gentleman." He had only one drink during dinner, as did you – a glass of wine each. At the end of the evening, he invites you in (or you invite him in) for a nightcap or a cup of coffee. You're both on the couch, chatting and enjoying good conversation. One thing leads to another and you start kissing. He starts moving a little too fast for your liking, and you say, "I'm not ready." He backs off. But 5 or 10 minutes later he starts up again. You say, "Stop!" But this time he overpowers you and does as he wants.

Example 2: You meet a guy at a beach party. Both of you have had too much to drink. He seemed nice when you met him and you thought he was attractive. But now that you've wandered off with him alone, he has plans. He's thinking that if your agenda fits his – great. However, if it doesn't, he knows he is going to do what he wants anyway. And there is virtually nothing you can do to stop him – no weapons, no people, just a guy who outweighs you by anywhere from 50 to 100 pounds.

Example 3: You and a girlfriend are walking home from a party late at night. (Younger girls, ages 12 to 15 are particularly susceptible to this.) Home is close enough that you can walk, but far enough that you're wishing you had a ride. A car with 2 or 3 guys pulls alongside, and they start chatting with you as you walk. You and your friend think they're cute. They seem nice. You're in a "good neighborhood." So when they offer to give you and your girlfriend a lift, you both figure, "Why not?" The two of you jump in, the driver spins the car towards the hills where he and his friends rape you both and leave you.

If these stories shake you up, they have served their purpose. Even though these are examples, they are real and happen every day. They have happened to women I have interviewed. More importantly, they have actually happened to your friends – whether you know it or not. 42% of rape survivors have never told anyone about the incident.[viii]

The *situational assailant*, by definition, rarely has a plan to attack a woman. He gets wound up by your beauty, alcohol, your outfit, a movie, or even a topic of conversation. Typically, you will have no clue or warning as to which action or event will bring about an attempted attack. It is extremely difficult to predict the trigger that will set this type of assailant into motion.

One of the few opportunities for recognizing a potential attacker exists in the early stages of a relationship. Listen to how he talks about women. Does he speak aggressively? Does he make derogatory comments about other people – male or female? None of these by themselves really matter or amount to much. The problem, once again, is that most dates (especially dinner dates) involve alcohol.

Alcohol is an accelerant. Most people think it is not. Alcohol magnifies a person's character traits – the good **and the bad**. A fun person becomes more fun. A sad person becomes more depressed. If a man is disrespectful, he becomes more so. If he is aggressive, this too steps up a notch. If he has not been with a woman for a while, his sense of need will magnify. These are not excuses for the behavior; they are warning signs. Approximately 75% of the men involved in acquaintance rapes had been drinking or using drugs just prior to the attack.[ix]

The later chapters that address dating and social gatherings offer tips about how to recognize the signs that things are going in the wrong direction. **ONCE A DATING SITUATION BEGINS HEADING IN THE WRONG DIRECTION, IT NEVER IMPROVES.** You must learn to recognize the warning signs as early as possible, and then remove yourself from this man's presence as quickly as you can.

The bottom line: remaining vigilant puts you in a greater position of power, in recognizing and avoiding both Serial and Situational Assailants.

Compact Discs of this book are available.
A © Copyrighted Scenario DVD
has also been produced.

Please visit the website listed below
to view or hear clips of the DVD or CD.

The website also has SPECIAL OFFERS
on multiple book purchases and bulk discounts
as well as information on
arranging public presentations.

www.**A World Without Rape**.org

Chapter Five

GHB the Date-Rape Drug

GHB (gamma-hydroxybutyrate or gamma hydroxybutyric acid) is the drug most commonly referred to as the "date rape drug." Its popularity has gone through the roof in recent years, especially on college campuses. It is now officially second only to Ecstasy as the "club drug" most frequently causing people to enter emergency rooms.

GHB is a man made product created by mixing a series of industrial agents (chemicals and solvents). It was originally marketed as an anesthetic and/or a sleep enhancer. It was banned by the FDA in 1990. Due to its widespread recreational use, GHB was categorized as a Schedule 1 controlled substance in March of 2000 by the DEA (Drug Enforcement Administration). Possession or distribution of a Schedule 1 controlled substance is a felony. Drugs such as heroin, cocaine, and meth-amphetamines are Schedule 1 drugs.

GHB is a powerful, fast-acting, central nervous system depressant. It does not produce a sense of euphoria, as many recreational drugs do. Low doses of GHB may cause short-term memory loss, sleepiness or giddiness. Larger doses can produce nausea, vomiting, headaches, delusions, hallucinations, drowsiness, dizziness, amnesia, respiratory problems, loss of muscle control, seizures, temporary paralysis, loss of consciousness and even death.

Because of their similarity to signs of intoxication, many of these symptoms can be confused by friends of a woman who's been drugged with GHB as the woman simply being drunk.

Since GHB is a synthetic product, the potency can be difficult to control. Also, oftentimes the drug is poured into a victim's drink in a hurried manner. This can also result in greater quantities of the drug being delivered to the recipient than the attacker may have intended.

GHB is odorless, colorless, and tasteless. It can be mistaken for water in both appearance and taste. Short of actually seeing someone put GHB into a woman's drink, there is virtually no way of detecting its presence. Also, GHB remains detectable in the blood system for only a limited period of time. If the victim is unaware that she was drugged or if aware, but waits too long to seek help or report the drugging, the opportunity to prove she was drugged is lost.

Some women have reported that GHB will have a salty or soapy taste. This IS possible since solvents are used in the production of GHB. However, when properly mixed, there is no ability to detect the presence of GHB in a drink or even in a glass of water. This being said, I address this for the primary reason that if a drink you have been drinking suddenly tastes "different" than it did a minute earlier or different than you know the drink *should taste*, **DO NOT finish the drink.**

Chapter Six

Awareness: Parking Lots, Cars and Public Transportation

PARKING LOTS

It doesn't just happen in the movies. The fact is: the vast majority of unknown assailant abductions take place in parking lots. Women's inattention to their surroundings and built-in preoccupations such as talking on cell phones, digging through a purse for car keys, not remembering where the car is parked, all contribute to making these sites welcome hunting grounds for predators.

Tip 1: Do not approach your vehicle if a paneled van or other large vehicle with darkly tinted windows is parked next to it. Find a security guard to walk you to your car; they are paid to do this. Even a nearby couple walking to their own vehicle can offer protection. Quickly say something like, "That vehicle wasn't here when I parked. Would you mind making sure I get into my car safely?" Most people, having been asked by a woman walking alone, would be happy to give 10 seconds to make sure she'll be okay.

IMPORTANT NOTE: Women are sometimes afraid to ask for assistance, out of fear that they may look foolish or be judged. Please err on the side of caution and **do not fall into this trap!** If I ever suspected that someone had broken into my home, even if I had a gun in my possession, I would still go to a neighbor's home and drag the police out to check on the situation. If I was wrong – oh well. I might be a little embarrassed, but ultimately there's no harm done.

If, on the other hand, I'm right and an intruder is in the home – I stay alive and uninjured. **You must learn to think the same way!**

Tip 2: If the parking lot is dark, is not normally well populated or if you know there have been problems in the area, ask to be escorted to your car by a security guard, co-worker, or other trusted individual.

Tip 3: Walk with purpose. (This will be a *recurring theme*.) Study after study has shown that a quick, purposeful walk sends subconscious signals to predators that you are not an easy target. They will usually decide to wait for another victim.

Tip 4: Pay attention to your surroundings. Look around. Make note of someone sitting alone in a car near yours or of a person or people hanging around near your car. If you see a person or group of people that could pose a potential threat, return to the store or office and ask to be escorted to your vehicle.

Tip 5: Keep one hand free at all times. This at least gives you the opportunity to attempt to fend-off a would-be attacker.

Tip 6: Have your key ready to open the door. **NEVER** stand next to your car searching your purse for your car keys. Robbers, car-jackers, and sexual predators all watch for this type of distraction. They wait for this moment to attack.

Tip 7: Once in your car, lock the doors **immediately.** This is the time when a bystanding predator you had not noticed, simply opens your car door and lets himself in. This happens frequently because it is such a quick and simple movement which attracts almost no attention from passersby.

Tip 8: Get your car moving. Get in motion immediately. Don't just sit in the vehicle adjusting the stereo, rummaging through your purse for your cell phone, or engaging in other activities – especially if the parking lot is not well populated. If you need to retrieve something from your bag, drive to a populated, well-lit area and stop the car (but leave it running) then search for the item.

APPROACHING YOUR VEHICLE AFTER SUNSET

Tip 9: Always be aware of your surroundings. Obviously, since it is dark, it is much more difficult to observe someone sitting in the car next to yours, or leaning against or behind a tree or other protrusion/obstruction. Have your key already in hand, ready to unlock your door. **NEVER** approach your vehicle if a single male is loitering anywhere near it.

Entering a vehicle is one of the most vulnerable moments for any person. If you have an alarm/locking button or keyless entry system, make sure you unlock only the driver's door. Most keyless systems allow you to unlock either the driver's door or by clicking twice, to unlock all doors. Unlocking all the doors permits a predator to simply get into your car from the passenger side. Once inside, he can do whatever he wants.

Tip 10: Make sure your dome light (interior light) is always functioning properly. As you unlock your vehicle and the interior illuminates, quickly glance into the back area to make sure an attacker has not already gained access to your car. If you do see someone, run to any populated area where you can call the police, giving them the make and location of your car. Try to remain in a position where you can see your vehicle, so that if the person gets out of the car, you can give his description to the police. However, do not sacrifice your own safety for getting the description.

Once you've checked the interior of your car, get in, lock the doors and get moving.

DRIVING ALONE IN YOUR VEHICLE

Tip 11: Always drive with your windows up and doors locked. If the windows must be down, make sure they are rolled up high enough that someone cannot easily reach in and open your door.

Tip 12: Service your car regularly. Keep a watchful eye on things like fan belts, hoses and fluid levels. Watch your gas gauge. Don't let your gas tank run below a quarter full.

Tip 13: Try to avoid deserted roads, especially at night. It is better to take the long way around than to run the risk of breaking down in the middle of nowhere.

Tip 14: If you run out of gas or break down during daylight, take the following steps: a) turn on your hazard lights; b) remain in your vehicle with the doors locked; c) do not accept a ride from a stranger. If someone stops to offer assistance, simply ask them to call a tow truck or the police.

Tip 15: If you run out of gas or break down **at night**, do the following: a) turn on your hazard lights; b) get out of the car and wait nearby in a well-lit, populated location; c) if there is no well-lit area nearby, or you are stuck in the middle of nowhere, turn on your hazards and hide in some bushes or behind a tree until help arrives. *Hit the Brakes on Car Repair Rip-Offs* gives a great deal of information about, not only avoiding being ripped-off, but also on maintaining your car so that it will perform in a safe manner thereby lessening the likelihood of breakdowns.

Tip 16: Make sure your spare tire has air in it. Also, carry a can of liquid air sealant for flat-tire repair. Most flat tires are the result of nails or other slow leak catalysts. These tire-sealing canisters also have a mechanism that refills your tire with air, permitting you to drive to a safe location. Drive to the nearest service station and have your bad tire replaced with your spare. These tire repair canisters only cost about $7 and can be purchased at any auto-supply or drug store.

Tip 17: If you carry a weapon, do not leave it in an unoccupied car. Leaving weapons in cars is one way we arm regular criminals. Further, if an assailant has acquired entry to your vehicle, he is now armed. (For additional information pertaining to weapons and their use, see Chapter 14, Thwarting an Attack.)

Tip 18: When entering a gated or secured parking garage, glance around the garage and make sure no one is loitering. Then stop your car and watch the gate close. The purpose of this practice is to ensure that someone is not following you in as the gate closes. Garages and secured parking structures present the perfect opportunity to predators and other criminals. These locations usually have low visibility and also alert attackers of the presence of others with bells and buzzers on gates, doorways and elevators. If you see someone who looks out of place or see someone run into the garage as the gate closes, leave the parking structure immediately and call the police. Do not assume that you will somehow be able to park, exit your car and get into your building before this person gets to you. Remain in your car, drive to a safe location, and call the police.

Tip 19: When leaving a gated or secured parking garage, stop your car just outside the gate or garage door and watch it close. Make sure no one has jumped inside as the gate or door is closing. Practice this habit consistently, as it benefits both you and your neighbors. If you do see someone run into the garage or parking structure as the gate or door closes, try to get a good look at the person, then call the police with a description.

Tip 20: If someone tries to flag you down while you are driving, look around. If it is clearly a bad situation, such as a bad accident, you may need to stop. If it is a single male, with his car parked to the side of the road, **DO NOT STOP.** Keep moving and call the police to report his location. If you don't have a phone, stop at the nearest public place and call 911. I understand not stopping may go against human nature, in that we often want to help others when we can, but you **absolutely** must place your personal safety before the inconvenience of another person.

Tip 21: If, while driving, the occupant of another car points to your car, acting as though something is wrong, do NOT stop **unless you become aware that something *really is* wrong.** An example of this might be a driver pulling alongside your car and pointing down at your car as though you have a flat tire.

You can feel a flat tire by the way a car is handling and you can look out your rearview mirror to see whether or not smoke is coming from the back of your car. If something does appear to be wrong, safely pull to the right side of the road, turn on your hazard lights, but do not get out of the car. If the driver of the other vehicle also pulls over, ask him to summon help. And be sure to thank him. **However,** do not accept a ride if one is offered. You have no way of knowing if this man has had anything to do with the problem your car is experiencing. If you do not believe anything is wrong with your car, **do not pull over.** Try to write down the other car's license plate number or the car's make, model, and color along with a description of the driver, then stop at the first public place available – gas station, fast food place, etc. Check to see if your car seems to be okay. If nothing appears to be wrong, alert the police with the information about the other driver.

Tip 22: If someone is following you, turn on your hazard lights and watch for a police officer or firefighters. If possible, drive to the nearest police or fire station. Many bars and clubs have uniformed police officers or off-duty officers working the front door. If you are unfamiliar with the neighborhood, it is sometimes easier to look for a bar or club rather than a police station. Remember that you can also use your horn to attract attention.

Tip 23: Keep your car key and house keys on separate rings. Parking attendants sometimes work in tandem with thieves or other criminals. Once they have your house keys, they can copy them for access at a later time. They can also have someone waiting at your home when you return. Or, knowing you will be out of the house for the next couple of hours, they can simply send someone to your home while you're having dinner.

Tip 24: While you are required by law to have your registration in your car, it does not have to be the original document. Make a copy of the registration, black-out the street address, then copy it again. Keep this copy in the car to present to law enforcement. Now, if someone breaks into your car or a parking lot attendant "likes what he sees," there is no way of tracking you back to your residence.

Tip 25: Do not leave any documents in your car with your address or social security number on them.

PUBLIC TRANSPORTATION

Tip 26: If you need to wait for public transportation, try to do so with other people. If there are no other people around, keep your back to the wall so that someone cannot sneak up on you from behind.

Tip 27: If riding public transportation, ride as close to the front of the bus or train as possible.

Tip 28: Do not fall asleep when riding a bus or train.

Tip 29: Watch who exits with you. If you have a bad feeling about the person, jump back on the bus or train and alert the driver.

Tip 30: If you disembark from a bus or train, and later see someone following you who was riding with you, quickly get to a well-populated area and call the police.

Chapter Seven

Awareness: While Walking or Jogging

Tip 1: Walk with speed and confidence at a quick, goal-oriented pace. Personal space and demeanor matter. Walk like you own the street. Most predators sense potential problems from women who walk in this manner.

If someone is walking in the opposite direction, look them straight in the face. Do not avoid eye contact. This may feel uncomfortable, but it reinforces to a predator that you are not afraid. Remember, stealth is the predator's most important operating method. He needs his victim to go quietly; drawing as little attention as possible. If your actions cause a potential attacker to think, "She will not go quietly," it's likely he'll make the decision to wait for an easier target.

Tip 2: If someone attempts to start a conversation with you, tell him you are late to meet your boyfriend or husband. Continue walking with purpose. You can be polite, while letting him know that you are not interested. Also, since this man does not actually know your destination, he will have no way of knowing if your "boyfriend" is a mere 30 feet off or a mile away. In this situation, the predator will usually keep moving, preferring to locate another victim. Do not stop walking to engage with this person. Again, even in emergency situations, most men are capable of understanding a single woman's reluctance to assist.

Tip 3: Do not wear earphones while walking or jogging. Do as much as you can to maintain a high level of awareness of your surroundings.

Tip 4: If possible, walk or jog with a friend or work associate. There is strength in numbers. Do not trail jog alone.

Tip 5: Try to avoid low-traffic areas or places populated with few people. It is far better to walk a few blocks out of your way than to put yourself at risk.

Tip 6: If you are ever approached by a man with a gun, **RUN!** It is very important to know that shooting a gun in real life is not like it appears in the movies. First of all, it is extremely difficult to hit a moving target. Second, guns attract a lot of attention. Additionally, the assailant is not interested in killing his victim, at least not at the time of initial contact. Thus, shooting his victim serves no purpose. Your running will usually cause the assailant to hightail it in the opposite direction.

If your assailant has a knife but is holding it away from your body, again: **RUN!** Remember, a knife is a close-quarter weapon. The quicker you can put distance between you and your attacker, the less purpose close-range weapons serve. Assailants use weapons to paralyze and intimidate potential victims. Most assailants, on the initial approach, have no desire to utilize a weapon; it is merely a tool to help them accomplish their end goal of robbery, kidnapping, sexual assault, etc.

Tip 7: Walk or jog opposite to the flow of traffic. Even if someone stops their car and displays a gun, you can quickly continue in the opposite direction of the traffic, making it very difficult for the attacker to do anything other than leave. Make sure you immediately report any incident of attempted violence or attack. Try to get the car's make and color or license plate. The police will respond quickly to these types of calls, especially if they think an attacker may still be in the area.

Tip 8: If you are walking or jogging and a vehicle pulls alongside you, watch for occupants other than the driver. NEVER approach a vehicle with multiple adult occupants. It only takes 2 seconds for a passenger to swing open a door and pull you in to the vehicle. Remain as far away from the vehicle as possible. If it is simply a single person wanting directions and you can give them without putting yourself at risk, go ahead. However, if there is any indication of a weapon or that something is out of line, **IMMEDIATELY MOVE** in the direction opposite the flow of traffic.

Tip 9: If you are walking or jogging and notice someone following you, cross the street and get to some place that's busy. If you notice you are still being followed, call the police.

Tip 10: Do not take shortcuts. Don't cut between buildings or through wooded areas just to shave 4 or 5 minutes off the time to your destination.

Tip 11: If you walk or jog regularly to and from work, to and from a bus stop, or on a regular exercise regimen, try to alternate your patterns either by varying your timing, your route, or both. And remember: it is best not to jog alone, especially on trails.

Tip 12: If you are visiting a new town or are in an unfamiliar area of town, carry a map and try to pre-plan your route. Looking lost sends a "victim signal" to predators.

Tip 13: NEVER hitchhike.

Tip 14: Avoid walking or jogging at night. Remember, however, that people are basically good. If you are walking or jogging through an unfamiliar area or a place that makes you feel uncomfortable, and you spot other people walking, just approach them and ask if they would mind if you walked or jogged with them for a few blocks. Most people will be happy to help you out. Again, don't feel foolish making this request. In this day and age, if someone were to approach me with such a request, I would have no problem both understanding and obliging.

Tip 15: Girls walking home from school should *always* walk with another person.
DO NOT ALLOW ANY ADULT MALE OR VEHICLE WITH MALE OCCUPANTS TO APPROACH YOU. Even if someone *really* needs assistance, they should not be looking to a young girl for help. They can get directions or find a phone by driving another block or two to a local business.

Tip 16: Trust your instincts. If you are walking and get a bad feeling, move away from the area, or stop and turn around. These internal alarms are usually God's way of letting you know you may be about to enter some type of harmful situation.

Chapter Eight

Awareness: At Bars, Clubs and Parties

Tip 1: If you are going out for the evening, try to go with friends. When you're out with friends, try to watch out for one another. Predators often watch for a woman sitting alone at a table while her friends are out on the dance floor. Of course, regular non-predatory guys will also approach this same woman. Remember, though, better safe than sorry. In any event, try not to split away from your group.

Tip 2: Arrange for your return travel **before** going out. Make plans in advance about what will happen if one of you decides to leave with someone you know or meet. Determine who will be the designated driver and make sure that whoever that person is, understands their responsibility to get everyone home safely.

Tip 3: NEVER leave your drink unattended. When getting up to dance or use the restroom, you have three options: 1) finish your drink; 2) take it with you; or 3) abandon it. Do not drink from a glass you have left unattended. It only takes a split-second to pour a vial of GHB into a glass. At that point, all the predator needs to do is sit back and wait for the drug to take effect. Even if you are just sitting and chatting, keep a napkin over your drink as an extra precaution.

Tip 4: Watch your bartender. While it's not a pleasant thought, it is possible the bartender may have a friend who has persuaded him to put something in your drink before it ever gets to you. **THIS ALSO HAPPENS IN SITUATIONS WHERE THE WOMAN HAS KNOWN THE BARTENDER.**

Tip 5: Watch alcohol intake – both yours and that of the people around you. As many as 55% of the women involved in acquaintance rapes had been drinking or using drugs just prior to the attack.[x]

SOME FACTS ABOUT ALCOHOL

- A 140-pound woman has less water in her body than a 140-pound man. This means a woman's blood alcohol level rises more quickly than a man's and the effects of the alcohol will last longer. Bottom line: women get drunk faster and remain drunk longer than men.

- Alcohol impairs everyone's judgment and their ability to think clearly. Things a man may say or do will look very different when you've had 2 or 3 drinks than they would if you were sober. When drinking, it becomes more difficult to notice the subtle behavior traits of a potential attacker.

- Alcohol impacts the men around you. If you do not know a man personally, you have no way of knowing which personality trait(s) the alcohol might magnify. As stated earlier, aggressive men become more aggressive, sexually charged men become increasingly so, etc.

Tip 6: Know the **difference** between *acquaintances* and *friends*. You have a male friend who is "like a brother" to you. You know, without question, this guy would never do anything to hurt you – drunk or sober. On the other hand, acquaintances are guys that seem nice enough; you may have hung out with them in a group a few times or bumped into them at the same parties or clubs, *but you don't REALLY know them.* I've lost track of the number of times a woman has told me, "I never would have expected *him* to have done this to me."

Tip 7: If you notice that one of your friends seems to have lost her motor skills (this is easily confused with being extremely drunk) and see a man offer to give her a ride, **YOU MUST TAKE CONTROL OF THE SITUATION AND MAKE SURE SHE GOES HOME WITH YOU.** I have heard countless stories about 4 or 5 buddies setting up a girl for a member of the group. These were usually men the women knew as acquaintances; men these women felt they could trust. I've seen these situations go both ways: times where a friend stepped in, removed her girlfriend from the situation, and drove her home; as well as times when no one did anything, allowing one of the acquaintance guys to drive the girl home only to have the "drive" turn into a rape or assault. Just because someone you've met seems nice, doesn't mean he is.

If you or your girlfriend has been drugged, the guy(s) offering the ride is/are almost always the perpetrators of the drugging.
DO NOT LET HIM/THEM TAKE YOU OR YOUR FRIEND HOME.

Compact Discs of this book are available.
A © Copyrighted Scenario DVD
has also been produced.

Please visit the website listed below
to view or hear clips of the DVD or CD.

The website also has SPECIAL OFFERS
on multiple book purchases and bulk discounts
as well as information on
arranging public presentations.

www.**AWorldWithoutRape**.org

Chapter Nine

Awareness: In Your Home or Apartment

Tip 1: You've just moved to a new home or apartment. Re-key all exterior locks. This will prevent former owners, renters or other keyholders from entering your residence without your permission.

Tip 2: Install a peephole in your front door. The person who re-keys your locks can do this at the same time.

Tip 3: Re-program your garage door opener. This is seldom mentioned, but your garage door is the quickest and least noticeable way to enter a home. Don't assume that your opener was the only unit floating around. There is usually a toll-free customer service number right next to the model number on both the hand-held control and the opener in your garage. Call the 800 number and ask them to walk you through the process of re-programming the unit. This precaution usually takes less than 3 minutes.

Tip 4: Do not hide spare keys around your property. Intruders know that many people engage in this practice and upon their approach, will quickly glance around for potential locations of hidden keys (e.g., the mailbox, above the door rim, under a planter, etc.) If you want a spare to be available for emergencies or lock-outs, leave a copy of your key with a trusted neighbor.

Tip 5: Your mailbox should not have your first name on it. Instead of "Barbara Smith," it should read "The Smiths." Technically, no name is necessary on a mailbox; the mail will still be delivered.

Tip 6: Do not throw phone bills, bank statements, credit card statements or other sensitive documents into the garbage without shredding them first. Something as seemingly innocuous as a phone bill gives a stalker or predator a complete list of all of your contact numbers (parents, family, friends, work, etc.) Shred or discard all sensitive documents in an appropriate manner

Tip 7: If your boyfriend had a key and you have broken up, change your locks. Even if your key was returned, you have no way of knowing whether or not a copy was made. If your boyfriend had a garage door opener, change the code. (Follow the steps in Tip 3.)

Tip 8: Most garages have standard interior doors that exit to a side yard. Make sure this door is bolt-locked. These doors are the MOST COMMON POINT OF ENTRY FOR INTRUDERS. If you are pulling into your garage and see this door open, **LEAVE IMMEDIATELY** and call the police.

Tip 9: When approaching your home, if there is any sign of an attempted entry (e.g., an open front door, open garage, open window that you know was closed, etc.), **do NOT enter the house.** Use your cell or go to a neighbor's to contact the police immediately. You have no way of knowing if the trespasser is still in the house. Do not assume that just because there is no foreign vehicle (a car you don't recognize) in the driveway that someone is not in your home.

Tip 10: Keep the bushes around your property trimmed – especially near doors and windows. This will make it more difficult for a potential attacker to hide.

Tip 11: Make sure the points of entry into your home or apartment and parking area are well lit. The best types of lighting systems are motion-activated floodlights. These are great because they don't burn electricity all night, yet the slightest movement lights up an entire area. You can purchase these at any hardware store. They are relatively easy to install wherever a light socket already exists.

If you live in a rental unit and the light is out at your front door, in the parking area, or any other dark location, report it. Landlords and property owners in virtually every state are required to provide minimum levels of safety assurance. Part of this duty involves ensuring that exterior lights are functioning properly.

Tip 12: If you believe someone is outside your home at night, **do not open your curtain to look outside.** Go into a different room that is dark and close the door behind you. Open a blind or drapery about an inch so you can get a view of your yard. Without a light on, it will be very difficult, if not impossible, for anyone to detect your presence. If you see a prowler, call the police. Even if you do not actually see a prowler, but suspect someone is lurking in your yard, still phone the police. As always – better safe than sorry.

Tip 13: A *serial assailant* may dress as a service or repair man or even as a police officer. Use the peephole to see who is at your door. Ask the person to hold their identification up where you can see it. Do not let someone inside your residence in order to check their identification. No legitimate visitor will have a problem with any of these requests.

If you are expecting a repairman, you can be reasonably assured he is who he says once he's shown his identification. If you are not expecting a repairman, dial 411 for information, get the phone number of the company, call that number and confirm the person is supposed to be there. **Do not call the number the person at the door gives you.** If you live in an apartment and the person at the door tells you something like, "The manager sent me to check on such and such," call your apartment manager to confirm the guy is supposed to be there. If you cannot confirm the information, **do not let him in.** If you find out he is not supposed to be there, call the police and try to provide as accurate a description as possible including approximate height, weight and the color and type of clothing he was wearing.

Tip 14: If you live alone and someone knocks on the door, as you approach the door, call out something like, "I've got it honey." Make sure you say this loud enough to be heard on the other side of the door. This will give the person at the door the impression there is someone else in the house. (Note: Technically you should always do this even if someone else really is home.)

Tip 15: You should never answer the door at night unless you are expecting someone. If you do answer, have your phone in your hand and as you approach the door say, "I've got it honey." **DO NOT** get talked into opening the door because of an "emergency" or for any other reason. If the person claims there is an emergency, tell the person, without opening the door, that you will phone the police for him or her.

Tip 16: Do not open your door just because you have a chain on it. A chain serves virtually no purpose and gives many people a false sense of security. It takes less than 15 pounds of pressure to force open a door that is "chain protected." In other words, *ANY* man, with virtually **ZERO EFFORT**, can force his way in through a partially open, chained door. Instead, if you have to open the door to check identification, receive a package, or for any other reason, put your foot behind the door and open it approximately 2 or 3 inches to the point where it is wedged against your foot. Three inches is plenty of room through which to pass an ID card, or see who is there; while it is not enough for a criminal to get his hand inside. If the person tries to push his way in, like you see in the movies, the door will bounce back at him, off your foot, and will pretty much close by itself. Bolt-lock the door and call the police immediately.

Tip 17: Do not let children answer the door. They are notorious for just swinging the door open. Even if you have trained them to ask who it is, if someone responds, "It's the police," your child will still probably open the door without confirmation.

Tip 18: Do not take showers, baths, or sleep with your doors unlocked or your sliding doors open. You are **completely defenseless** while engaged in these activities.

Tip 19: Your listing in the phone book should not have your first name or your address. We see listings all the time for "B. Smith." The problem is: this is a pretty good indicator of a female living alone. You have a few choices. Have the listing read "Barbara and Paul Smith" (even though there is no Paul) or "B & P Smith." If neither of these options appeals to you, go ahead and use "B. Smith," but exclude your address. List your city only.

Tip 20: If someone calls and you are unsure as to who it is, put your hand over the phone (lightly) so the person on the other end can still hear you, and say, "I'm on the phone honey." You do not want unknown callers or visitors thinking you are home alone. Do not engage in phone conversations with people you do not know. Never give out personal information over the phone.

Tip 21: Know that your cordless phone can be eavesdropped on. Cordless phones operate on radio frequencies, and virtually any scanner can pick up your conversation. Do not have private conversations on cordless phones. If you are planning on having a confidential conversation, use a landline. A landline is a phone which has the cord attached to the dialing unit, which is then plugged in at the wall.

Tip 22: If you have been receiving prank/stalker type calls, you have a few options:

Option 1: Some people suggest keeping a whistle next to the phone, and if the perpetrator calls back a second or third time, blow the whistle into the mouthpiece. I am not a fan of this because I think it could anger a caller. However, some reports confirm this practice does work – especially with 2 am *drunk dialers*.

Option 2: Hang up. Then dial *69 and hang up when the phone is picked up. This is an automatic redial feature on most home or apartment phones. You will not be able to see the redialed number, but once redialed, the phone company has a record of the number, thereby enabling the police to track down the caller. This feature does not work on every call nor on calls originating from cell phones.

Option 3: If the calls lead you to believe someone is watching you or your home, call the police immediately. New technologies exist that permit instantaneous tracing of certain calls.

Tip 23: Close your curtains or blinds at night. Even something as simple as illumination from a television is enough to "fishbowl" an entire room.

Tip 24: If you live in a house or large apartment, turn on lights in two different rooms at night. This gives the impression that more than one person is home. A predator is much more likely to attempt an attack if he thinks a woman is alone.

Tip 25: Install a lock on your bedroom door and make sure you have a phone in the bedroom. **If you believe someone is in your home, DO NOT exit your room to investigate.** Instead, with your phone in your hand, stand at your door and listen. If you confirm someone is in the house, quickly call the police. Intruder calls are *immediate response* calls. Law enforcement responds faster to these calls than virtually all others.

Tip 26: Test all your window and door locks to ensure they are functioning properly.

Chapter Ten

Awareness: In Offices, Elevators and Stairways

Tip 1: If you must be in an office after dark, make sure the doors are locked. If you are expecting people, let them know ahead of time the door will be locked, and they should call you to let them in.

Tip 2: Do not open an office door to someone you do not know. In an office environment, there is often no one around to help you if you become the victim of an after-hours attack.

Tip 3: When leaving an office at night, ask someone to walk you to your car. Parking lots are the primary locations for abductions and attacks. If no one is available, have your key in hand, walk with purpose, check the area as you approach your car, check the back seat, get in, lock the doors, and get the car in motion as quickly as possible.

Tip 4: If using an elevator, check the elevator before entering. If there is already someone in it, and you get a bad feeling about the occupant, wait for the next car.

Tip 5: If waiting for an elevator, notice your surroundings. Does there seem to be someone just hanging around who could quickly rush into the elevator as the doors close?

Tip 6: Upon entering an elevator, stand toward the front, as close to the control panel as possible. If something goes wrong, you can hit the alarm button or press all the buttons. Pressing all the buttons will force the elevator to stop at each floor, increasing the odds of someone entering the elevator or giving you a chance to get out. If an attacker chases after you from the elevator, as you run through the corridor try to spot a fire alarm on the hallway walls and pull the lever. **Everybody responds to fire alarms.** Your attacker will immediately flee the scene.

Tip 7: It is generally not a good idea for a woman to use a sealed interior staircase, unless it is located in a well-trafficked office building.

Chapter Eleven

Awareness: On Job Interviews

This section deals more with modeling and acting interviews than standard job interviews. Sexual assault stories that appear in major media markets such as Los Angeles and New York, may not make their way into other states or even smaller communities within the same state.

Young women, roughly between 16 and 25, fall prey to the situations described in this chapter. The scenario looks something like this: A man walking through a mall, or other well-trafficked area, approaches a woman while she's shopping or out with friends. He says he's late for an appointment, but that he is a talent scout, or other party engaged in locating models or actresses, and that he would like your phone number to contact you for an interview/audition. While this person may truly be some type of talent scout or agent, you need to take the same precautions you would with any other stranger. Oftentimes these individuals turn out to be *serial assailants*. It is not unusual to read or hear about their victims in news stories telling of how some young woman disappeared after going out for a job interview but was later found dead with signs of sexual assault.

The following will help to keep you aware of situations that can place you at risk.

Tip 1: Never give out your phone number to a stranger. Ask the person for *their* phone number and tell them you will call them.

Tip 2: When calling the number for the first time – even if you were given a business card, call the number from a blocked phone line during regular business hours (8 am to 5 pm). If no-one answers, hang up. Any legitimate business will have someone answering the phones. If your phone rings immediately after hanging up do not answer it – you have just been *69'd.

If you are calling an 800 number, the only phone that will register "unknown caller" is a blocked cell phone. Calls originating from land lines, even when blocked, are displayed on "caller id" when dialing 800 numbers.

It is not unusual for private citizens and small companies to NOT answer calls from blocked numbers. If you are calling a small company from a blocked number, you may end up in voicemail or an automated answering system. Listen to the answering device. If the message goes anything like this, "Hey. You've reached Tony. Leave a message." DO NOT LEAVE A MESSAGE. Bona fide talent scouts and agents give business cards with land line telephone numbers that are usually answered by a live person – whether or not someone is calling from a blocked number. This man may not be a sexual predator, but he is probably not who he claims to be.

Tip 3: If it is requested that you come in for an interview, screen test or any other type of audition:

- Check the company before going to the appointment. Go to an online search engine such as Yahoo!® and type in the company name. Almost every *real* company has a website. If no website shows up or if there are negative blogs regarding the company, cancel the appointment.

- Do not set any appointment for any time other than a weekday during daylight. There are some companies that run weekend auditions to make it easier for teenagers; this is okay.

- NEVER go to an appointment without a friend or family member accompanying you. Legitimate companies completely understand a young woman's need to ensure her safety. They might ask that your friend remain in a waiting area during the interview; this would be a reasonable request.

Tip 4: Do not leave the meeting location to travel to another site unless accompanied by a male friend or family member.

Tip 5: Do not leave your purse, keys or cell phone unattended.

Tip 6: If this is your first interview with a company and you are called by someone saying they represent the organization and the caller tells you the meeting location has been changed, cancel the appointment. It is very rare that a legitimate company will send you out for an audition without having first interviewed you at their own offices.

Tip 7: If after interviewing with a company you are sent to a location for an audition, interview or shoot, always take an adult male with you. If the location is a legitimate site with plenty of people around, you can ask your companion to wait in the car. If, however, you have any uneasy feeling about the location or the people who are there, ask your friend or family member to accompany you inside.

Do not be embarrassed by how you *might look* by bringing someone with you. "Industry" people know that women need to take precautions.

To summarize: any legitimate scouting agent should have offices in a professional environment. And this would be the location for your first appointment or interview. **Do not meet anywhere else.**

Chapter Twelve

Awareness: Online Dating Sites

Internet dating has added a new dimension to sexual assault. Many people feel that online dating is dangerous. And while you should still follow certain rules, online dating is actually one of the safest methods of meeting people.

The reason for this high level of safety is the electronic trail left through dating communications. This trail is usually enough to deter *serial assailants*. First, there is the process of signing up to join an online dating service. Credit cards are almost always required. A credit card obviously has a name and current address associated with the card. So any type of serial predator knows that any illegal activity (such as rape or sexual assault) will bring about rapid identification and apprehension. Predators do their best to operate below the radar and would almost never use their own credit card to join an online dating service. And, unlike the ease of setting up a fake email, using a fake or stolen credit card for online dating has virtually no appeal to the bad guys.

The next stage of the electronic trail is email. Since your communications through online dating services begin with email, there is always an email account that can be traced. While there are temporary email services that enable people to acquire an email address only to ditch the address 10 minutes later, this holds no value in online dating situations where back and forth communications can easily span hours, days or even weeks. Temporary email services do not enable extended back and forth communication.

Email addresses, even those such as Yahoo!® or Hotmail® can still be tracked to a specific IP address. IP stands for *internet protocol*. An IP address can be traced to a specific computer at a specific location. This too dissuades predators from using online dating sites as "hunting grounds."

The final aspect of the electronic trail is the phone number. Since almost 100% of meetings are confirmed by phone, the perpetrator (or potential perpetrator) of a crime can now be tracked down by his phone number as well.

So, in actuality, it is far easier for a *serial assailant* to walk into a bar, leave with a woman and commit a crime against that woman without any person ever being able to identify him than it is to commit assaults through online dating services.

This being said, a woman still needs to be aware of *situational assailants* as discussed in Chapter 4 and there are still a number of safe practices that can decrease a potential bad date scenario. And remember, just because a date is bad, does not mean the guy is a sexual predator. But who wants to waste time and energy on a bad date?

The following are suggestions that can help avoid online dating disasters while maintaining your safety.

Tip 1: Do not use any online dating service that does not require a credit card. Without verification through the use of a credit card, you have no way of knowing who you are about to meet and the police may have a difficult time in tracking the person should something happen to you.

Tip 2: No Photo = No Contact. It is understandable that certain people desire privacy, but the "rules" of online dating say that if you are going to engage, you should post a photo. **ALWAYS require a photo prior to agreeing to meet someone.** You need to have some way of identifying who you are meeting – other than, "I'll be the guy holding a rose."

Some people might say, "What's to stop someone from posting someone else's picture?" The answer is – nothing. But either you will recognize the guy when he shows up, or you will not. If he does not look like the guy in the ad posting, don't engage UNDER ANY CIRCUMSTANCES. No matter how nice or good looking he might seem, odds are this person is a predator. Get to a crowded area as quickly as possible and call a friend for a ride or ask for a manager to escort you to your car. Whatever you do, do NOT leave the meeting place alone.

Tip 3: If a man's dating profile pictures make him unrecognizable, I would suggest passing on the profile. Dark glasses, hats, pictures taken at a distance are all signs that a guy is trying to hide something – be it age, lack of hair or even his identity. While there could be a multitude of reasons for this practice, **none of these reasons have *any* benefit to you.**

Tip 4: If a man's profile shows frequent drinking or any drugging habits (e.g. "420 friendly"), just remember that roughly 60% of all sexual assaults take place where the victim, the perpetrator or both have been drinking or drugging.

Tip 5: Look for stability in the profile. Simple things like jobs, family and friends are all good things for normal people to have. While it is very easy to lie in a profile, you can gather or confirm vital information just by paying attention during your pre-meeting emails or phone contacts. For example: If you're receiving communications during working hours it is possible the guy is unemployed. Is an unemployed guy a bad guy? Not necessarily. Do you want to pay for your dates to Top Dog or McDonalds®? Probably not.

Tip 6: At such point in time that you agree to leave the dating service email format and exchange personal email addresses make sure that your full name is not in your address. It is not unusual to see Mary.Smith@sbcglobal.net or something similar. Do not do this. Leave your last name off your email address. Actually, it is best to establish a Yahoo® or Hotmail® account for dating purposes. This way if you end up being harassed or cyber-stalked, you can just cut the email address loose and set up a new account.

Tip 7: When it comes time to exchange phone numbers, it is better to give out a cell number rather than a home number. Creative people can find out where you live by having access to your home number. You can always change your cell number if any type of harassment takes place.

Tip 8: Be aware of unusual area codes. If somebody gives you a phone number that includes an area code that you do not recognize, go to Yahoo!® and type in, "702 area code" and see what comes up. If the city associated with someone's number is not local to your region, your guard level should increase.

Setting up the meeting:

Tip 9: Once you've exchanged a few email or phone conversations and you feel comfortable about meeting, try to set up a daylight meeting in a public place. Meeting for coffee is usually best. There is an unstated expectation that you will not be spending an extended period of time when meeting for coffee. If you enjoy his company, you can always decide to grab a bite to eat. But, if the guy turns out to not be your type or you get an uneasy feeling, you can usually come up with some reason to leave after 20 or 30 minutes without appearing rude.

If you set a meeting at a coffee shop or some similar establishment, do NOT make it a place you frequent. Choose a location that is on neutral ground. If the guy you meet is not a match (and odds are he won't be) you don't want him showing up at your regular hangout in the hopes of "bumping into you."

Tip 10: If the man who shows up is anyone other than the guy in the photo, get someone at the establishment to escort you to your car and leave ASAP. If you walked to the location, call a friend to pick you up – do not walk home or back to work. I cannot stress this point enough. NEVER engage with someone who is not the person in the profile – no matter what the excuse or story. This person is a predator.

There are a few things you should do before leaving for any blind- or internet-generated date.

Tip 11: Print a copy of the photo or the dating profile of the person you are meeting and leave it on your desk, kitchen countertop or bed. Write the person's email address, phone number, and location you are meeting on the printout.

Tip 12: Tell a friend: the name of the guy you are meeting, his email and phone number and when and where you are meeting. Let's say you're meeting this person at 7 for drinks and/or dinner. Tell your friend that if they do not hear from you by 10pm to call the police. If you don't want your friend to "over-react" by calling the police, have your friend call you or give your friend a quick update call or text just letting them know that everything's kool. (You don't have to be rude about this call in front of the person you're with, just inform your date that a friend asked you to check-in if too many hours passed. Any decent person should understand this precaution.)

If you decide to extend the date by staying out with this guy, call or text your friend and tell him or her that everything's okay and that you've decided to extend the date or that you won't be coming home and you will talk to them in the morning. Note: Make sure you review pages 76-84 which discusses returning to your place or his – neither of which is advisable on a first date.

Tip 13: Be sure to reread pages 71-75. These pages cover standard "blind- or internet-date" rules.

Online dating can be fun. Just be sure you take the proper precautions. No amount of information in a dating profile will answer the most important question about a guy – whether or not he can be trusted.

Chapter Thirteen

Awareness: Dating and Date Rape

In 80% of all rapes and sexual assaults, the victim knows her attacker. **80%!** That's 4 out of 5 cases! Recent statistics show this number moving closer to 90%.[xi]

In fully 50% of those attacks, the assault takes place in either the victim's or the perpetrator's residence. On college campuses, 60% of all attacks take place in the woman's residence.

In the majority of these situations, the sexual assault takes place early in the relationship timeline, meaning, it is more likely that a woman will be sexually assaulted within the first 2 or 3 dates, than in the ensuing 10. What this tells us is that women need to pay extra attention in the early stages of a relationship.

Remember, the Date Rape perpetrator usually falls under the *situational assailant* category (see pages 22-25). His actions are dictated more by what is going on in the moment than a clearly planned attack strategy. GHB-related assaults (also known as drug-facilitated assaults) generally are not included in the profile of a *situational assailant* since, by definition, the *situational assailant* has not preplanned an assault. However, this being said, GHB could be used in a date rape situation, by a perpetrator who is "tired of waiting" but unwilling to give up or take "no" for an answer.

There are a number of situations that can lead to date rape. We'll begin with the most basic and build to the more complex. We will also address actions you can take that may prevent a potential assault.

YOUR FRIENDS SET YOU UP WITH SOMEONE THEY KNOW (blind or semi-blind date)

Let's say you associate with a group that is generally more sexually active than you. They set you up with someone, or someone familiar with the group contacts you. This man may assume you have the same sexual habits/values as the rest of the group.

Tip 1: Establish your boundaries right up front. There are a couple ways to handle this.

a)   You can address the issue head-on.

Example: "Before we go out, I need you to know that some of my friends tend to be more sexually active than I. While I am not judging them, I want you to know that I believe in taking time to get to know someone." Then, define what you mean by "time." **Guys are not smart when it comes to this.** They might assume "time" to mean 2 and ½ hours. Spell it out and make it clear for them. "I believe in remaining celibate until marriage." Or, "I don't make out on the first date." Whatever your boundaries, make them known.

b)   You can address the issue in an off-handed manner.

Example: You're both just chatting, and you subtly mention that some of your friends move a little faster than you prefer. **The only problem with subtlety is that guys are not that smart,** and we (yes, me too) do not always get subtle hints. Quite often, we need to be hit in the head with a baseball bat. The up-front approach (as mentioned in "a" above) is usually the better method in dealing with this situation.

INTERNET DATE

No matter how you meet someone, you always have an opportunity to set clear boundaries. Again establish them up front. Tell the guy on the phone or through an e-mail prior to the meeting. That way, there can be no misunderstanding on the man's part. If he's looking for sex on the first date and you make it clear that you're not interested, you've just saved yourself a lot of grief – and a possible attack.

Tip 2: Make sure to tell someone you're going on an internet or blind date. Give your friend the phone number of the guy you will be meeting. If you decide to go back to his place and spend the night, call your friend and let them know.

Whether an internet date or a blind or semi-blind acquaintance date, try to do the following:

Tip 3: Drive YOUR OWN car to the meeting place. There are several reasons for this:

- You do not yet know the guy you're meeting. Therefore you cannot know if he has a drinking problem, and you do not want to depend on a drunk driver to get you home safely.

- The guy you're meeting may turn out to be not "your type." Therefore, having him know where you live is probably not the best idea.

- If things start to turn sour during dinner, you can leave without worrying about how you'll be getting home.

- If you do decide to go back to his place (which I do not advise), you can follow him in your own car. If when you get there, you have a bad feeling or sense that something is just not right, or if things start to get out of control inside his place, you can leave.

Tip 4: Try to meet your date in a public place. Don't agree to meet in some far-off, hard-to-reach, or secluded location. Again, there are a number reasons for this:

- You could get lost reaching the meeting place.

- You could get lost on your way home.

- You could be putting yourself at risk by entering an area where you are unaware of the locations of safety services, gas stations, etc.

Try to stick to a nice restaurant or venue close to your home or in an area that is familiar to you.

Tip 5: Watch your date. There are a number of things to watch for when meeting someone new.

1) First and foremost: Is he drinking more alcohol than you would prefer? Think about this: a man is driving to dinner or a club, then drinking too much – even when he *knows* he will have to drive himself and/or his date home. **This tells you a great deal about his**

priorities and the importance he places on other people – including YOU. If your date is more than willing to put you or other people on the road at risk, what will his thought process be if you ever find yourself in a position where you have to say "No"? Three drinks over the span of a 2-hour dinner will render the average man legally drunk – whether or not he is acting like it.

2) Pay close attention and assess how your date speaks about (and to) other people – especially women. If he speaks in a derogatory manner about his ex or others, you know that with some alcohol streaming through his system, these types of comments and attitudes will only get worse. Does your date make reckless or uncaring comments about friends, acquaintances, or people in general? Again, this is the sign of a person who does not have a lot of regard for others. A man who has little regard for others is unlikely to listen to your specific requests to "stop" when you're back at his place.

3) **NEVER** leave your drink unattended. You do not know this man yet. Acquaintance rapes make up 80% of all rapes and sexual assaults. Do not assume that just because your friends like him or think he's a nice guy, that he really is okay. Until you've been out with a guy 4 or 5 times, you really know **very little** about him. If you're on date at a restaurant or bar and need to use the restroom, ask the waiter for a fresh drink when you return.

THINGS CAN ONLY GET WORSE. Let me say that again. **THINGS CAN ONLY GET WORSE.** You will be hearing this line several times throughout this section.

Example: You are out for drinks, then dinner. Your date has had 2 or 3 drinks in the bar and he orders another couple of drinks during dinner. He is now officially drunk. (He also, most likely has a drinking problem.) If you have matched him, round for round, you are also drunk. His aggression level is now way up and your defenses are limited. With both of you in this state, the odds are dramatically increased that something will go very wrong. Call a friend or a cab and get yourself home.

Example: While speaking with you, your date touches your arm or leg, in a way that makes you uncomfortable. You, in response, either pull back or ask him to stop. He, in turn, pulls closer or does not stop the touching. Any man who, in public, repeatedly ignores a simple request to not violate your personal space will have absolutely no qualms about ignoring the request when the two of you are alone.

Example: You are out for drinks, then dinner. Your date initiates a conversation that you believe to be inappropriate this early in the relationship. You tell him you'd rather change the subject, which he does. Ten to 15 minutes later, he returns to the same inappropriate or offensive subject matter. You tell him again that you're not comfortable with the subject. But during dinner, he brings it up again. Obviously, this man does not care about your feelings. What do you think he'll be like when you're alone with him?

In any of the above 3 examples, it is better that your date think that you "just can't relax" or that you're a "prude," rather than allowing him to set the mental and physical tone for the remainder of the evening – which could very easily turn into a sexual assault.

BACK TO HIS PLACE (or yours)

Dinner was nice and you trust him enough to follow him back to his place. If you've already been drinking, out comes more alcohol (or the offer of same), guaranteed! At some point, he makes an aggressive move, letting you know that he wants the physical part to either get started or go further. If this is more than you want, you must use your hand, push his chest and say, "If you continue, I will leave." If his response is anything to the effect of, "Don't be so uptight" or any continuation of the physical behavior you are attempting to thwart, LEAVE without looking back. **THINGS CAN ONLY GET WORSE.**

Do not think you will be able to calm him down or handle the situation if things start to go wrong. The more sexually wound up he is, the less likely you will be able to stop his advances.

ON SELF-DEFENSE TECHNIQUES

I want to spend a minute here on the subject of self-defense. Let's say you have been taking self-defense classes or kick-boxing at your local gym. You feel good and you feel strong. This is not to demean your skills or athleticism, but I must issue a WARNING.

> **Example:** Fighter A and Fighter B have equal skill. The fighter with a 10- or 15-pound weight advantage will win virtually every time.

> **Example:** Fighter A is a better fighter than Fighter B. Fighter B weighs 25 or 30 pounds MORE than Fighter A. Fighter B will still likely win, due simply to his weight advantage.

Example: Fighter A is a way better fighter than Fighter B. Fighter B outweighs Fighter A by 60 or 80 pounds. The chance of Fighter A winning is almost zero, even though he is a MUCH more skilled fighter. **No matter what you know, how well you have mastered what you have learned, or how great of shape you are in, YOU ARE FIGHTER A.** It is highly unlikely that you will be able to physically overpower a man weighing 50 or more pounds than you.

As we discussed earlier, the average man weighs approximately 45 pounds more than the average woman. The chance of a woman being able to fend off an attack, without a weapon, is very low. Men are raised to fight. We begin wrestling with our fathers and friends as early as age 5, age 3 if we have older brothers. We watch and absorb fight scenes in movies, video games, and on television. Yet any man would still have a very difficult time overpowering another man who had a 45-pound weight advantage.

We are talking about your safety. You put yourself at risk when you operate under the assumption that you are capable of physically gaining the upper hand against a man, especially one outweighing you by 50 or more pounds. You, in fact, are putting yourself at risk simply by believing that you can handle whatever comes your way. It is not demeaning to assume that the man you're with will be able to overpower you. Operating under this mindset will prevent you from placing yourself at unnecessary risk.

BACK TO YOUR PLACE

Dinner was enjoyable. You both had a nice time. What next? You may be inclined to invite him back to your residence.

THE ADVANTAGES (of returning to your place)

- You are familiar with your own environment.

- You have good neighbors, and if you have to scream, you know someone will respond.

- You won't be put in the position of having to be the one who leaves. Since it's your place you can order him to get out.

THE DISADVANTAGES

- He now knows where you live.

- He now knows where you park your car.

- He now knows how to get into your building.

- He now knows whether or not you live alone. If you have housemates, he may not know, but can quickly learn, their patterns, because you will tell him, when he asks, "Where are your roommates?"

- He knows the physical layout of your home or apartment: the access points, where the phone(s) is/are, the quality of your locks, the nature of your neighbors, etc.

- He knows that just because a woman raises her voice does not mean the neighbors will come running. (As a rule, most neighbors do not want to get involved in what they will likely view as a domestic dispute situation.)

- He knows that you are not strong enough to overpower him.

- He knows that you probably have alcohol around the house, so even though it's not his own place, he can still manage to get both of you drinking.

BACK TO HIS PLACE

Dinner was enjoyable. You both had a nice time. What next? You may be inclined to go back to his place.

THE ADVANTAGES (of going back to his place)

- He does not learn where you live or anything about your lifestyle (e.g., whether it's an apartment or a house, whether you live alone or not, whether you have a dog, etc.)

- Sometimes leaving is easier than trying to force someone out.

THE DISADVANTAGES

- He has "home court advantage."

- He controls the alcohol or other liquids.

- He controls the phones.

- If he has locked the door and you try to get out quickly because the date has taken a turn for the worse, you may not be able to exit as quickly as you might need to.

- You may have set down your purse or keys. Again, if you have to leave quickly, you now have to collect your things.

Do the *Disadvantages* seem to outnumber the *Advantages*? In both scenarios?? They should! Because they do! **Whether it's his place or yours, returning to such a private location, puts you at risk.**

If you would like some quiet time with a new guy, go somewhere a little less busy than a restaurant, but still busy enough that you are not secluded. Remember, you only met this guy a few hours ago, or maybe a date or two ago. You still do not know him very well. It usually takes at least 4 or 5 dates to get to know someone's operating methods, and distinguishing whether the core set of beliefs they say they have actually lines up with their actions. For the first few dates, try to be somewhere at least semi-public.

BACK TO HIS PLACE – PRECAUTIONS

1) Use the restroom just as you leave the restaurant, club or bar. It is better to not use the bathroom in his home, unless absolutely necessary. Using his bathroom takes you out of the room that likely contains your drink, purse, phone, etc.

2) Drive yourself in your own car. If you arrive and don't like the situation, you can leave without waiting for someone to come and give you a ride.

3) Leave any personal items in your car, with the exception of your keys and possibly your cell phone. If you have to get out of his place quickly, you won't be preoccupied worrying about grabbing a bunch of different items.

4) Pay special attention to details as you enter his place. a) Most importantly – know his address. As you drive up to his place, you might just make a quick call a send a quick text to a friend and tell him/her your location - even if you just leave it on a voicemail. b) Make note of security gates, garage doors, foyers, etc. c) Look around and try to spot fire alarm levers. (Most every apartment and condominium building has them.)

Fire alarms are the single quickest way to get neighbors out of their apartments/condos and to summon help – a lot of help.

5) Look around the grounds and notice how you enter from and exit to the street. This is important even for less sinister events, such as fires or natural disasters.

6) Once inside his place, make a mental note of the locks on his door and watch how he closes it behind him. If you have to leave quickly, you will remember if the door was locked or chained.

7) Even if you are carrying your cell phone, look around for a phone. Your cell phone may not get clear reception. Also, cell calls to 911 are more difficult to trace than calls originating from land lines. There are times when it may be easier to grab a phone and retreat to a bathroom or bedroom and wait for help to arrive than it would be to actually try and escape through the front door. This is especially the case in the event of drug facilitated attacks.

8) Look around his place for anything that could be used as a weapon in the event he attempts an attack. Fireplace utensils, a baseball bat, or mid-size lamps are all easy to handle and can be swung at your attacker in a manner

that can produce injury. Knives or other close-quarter weapons should only be used as a last resort, and then used more to attempt escape rather than for combat. (See Chapter 14, Thwarting an Attack.)

9) Remember, it's his place. He is in control of **all** beverages. If you have not known this guy for very long, only accept drinks from closed, sealed containers. It is possible that he spiked a drink with GHB or some other depressant, before he even left his place for the date.

10) Watch *your* alcohol intake. The more drunk you are, the more difficult it will be to fend off an attack.

11) Watch *his* alcohol intake. Most men, even the most sedate, become more aggressive while under the influence of alcohol.

12) It is generally not a good idea to enter his bedroom early on in a relationship. The presence of a woman in a man's bedroom sends out a signal to him that you may be willing to have sex with him. **It does not matter whether or not you intend to send this signal.** All that matters is this is how your actions may be interpreted. Restrict your movements to the main living areas of the home or apartment.

13) Last but not least, remember, **THINGS CAN ONLY GET WORSE.** If something is starting to go wrong, your date is not suddenly going to become less drunk or less aggressive. **YOU NEED TO GET OUT.** Do not try to calm yourself by thinking, "I can handle this." Unless you are carrying a gun, and you probably are not, odds are you will not be able to thwart an attack.

BACK TO YOUR PLACE – PRECAUTIONS

1) Use the restroom just as you're leaving the restaurant, club or bar. It is better to not use the bathroom once you're home, unless absolutely necessary. If he is carrying some type of drug with him, you have no way of knowing whether or not he slipped it into your drink while you were out of the room.

2) Know where the fire alarms are in your building. In the event of an attack it may be easier to run out of your living area and into a corridor that would be quickly crowded by neighbors if a fire alarm lever is pulled.

3) Watch *your* alcohol intake. The more drunk you are, the more difficult it will be to fend off an attack.

4) Watch *his* alcohol intake. Most men, even the most sedate, become more aggressive while under the influence of alcohol.

5) Keep a phone in your bedroom and have a lock on the door.

6) Consider keeping a container of pepper spray near an access point, such as the transition between the kitchen and the living room, or the medicine cabinet in the bathroom – someplace where if you were trying to evade an attacker, you could grab the container while on the run.

7) It is generally **NOT** a good idea to invite a man into your bedroom early on in a relationship. Inviting a man into your bedroom sends out a signal to him that you're considering having sex with him. **It does not matter**

that you are not intentionally sending this signal, only that this is how he may be interpreting your actions. Also, attacks taking place in the bedroom are difficult to thwart, due to the limited mobility the environment provides. From a living room, you're more likely to be able to escape to the front door, the kitchen, a bedroom, or a bathroom. From a bedroom, you usually can only get to the door of the bedroom or to a bathroom. In the early stages of your relationship, it's best to restrict your socializing to the main living areas of the home or apartment.

8) Last but not least, remember, things can only get worse. If something is starting to go wrong, your date is not going to suddenly become less drunk or less aggressive. **You need to act quickly.** Throw him out! If that means picking up the phone and calling the police, then do so. Do whatever it takes to get him to leave.
THINGS CAN ONLY GET WORSE.

Purchase additional copies for your friends' daughters.

Purchase additional copies for your nieces.

Purchase additional copies for your neighbors' daughters.

Go to www.**VerumPress**.com

Together, we can end rape in America.

Chapter Fourteen

Thwarting an Attack

This section tackles possible scenarios in order of the greatest likelihood of an attack to the least. I will begin with social situations and end with street assaults.

DRUGGING SCENARIO 1: You are in a bar and are starting to feel strange. You have only had 1 or 2 drinks and should not feel the way you do. **DO NOT make the mistake of thinking you will feel better.** If you are with friends **immediately tell them** you think you may have been drugged and that you need them to get you to a hospital. If you are not with friends (*real friends*), find a police officer (most clubs now have on- or off-duty police officers working the front door), a bouncer or manager and tell him/her you think you may have been drugged. **Whatever you do, DO NOT ALLOW a male acquaintance, or a guy you just met, to take you home or to the hospital. This is most likely the person who drugged you.**

DRUGGING SCENARIO 2: You are at a party and begin noticing that you feel strange. Again, do not hope it will pass. Get to a girlfriend immediately and tell her that she needs to take you home or to the hospital. If she takes you home, make sure someone stays with you. If you have been drugged, you may simply fall asleep, however, depending on the drug, you could also slip into a coma. If you believe you or one of your friends has been drugged, the safest and smartest thing to do is to get to an emergency room. This is the only way to ensure your/their safety.

KNOWN ASSAILANT ATTACK SCENARIO 1:
You are at his place **and have just realized that you've been drugged.** Grab a phone, then run and lock yourself in a bathroom or bedroom. It is generally easier to get to one of these rooms, rather than trying to escape, especially since you don't know what kind of drug has been administered or how quickly you might become incapacitated. Even if you could get to your car, you would be unable to drive without putting yourself or others at risk. Dial 911. **Do not hang up** – even if you are placed on hold. If you cannot speak, a police unit will still respond to the location. These are known as "off-hook" calls and are usually interpreted by the police department as emergency situations. The police respond accordingly. The 911 emergency response system cross references phone company records to bring up the address associated with a non-cell telephone (land line). If there is a window in the bathroom, break it and yell out the window, "FIRE! Please help my baby." Do NOT waste time trying to figure out how to open a window. Grab any heavy object and break the glass. You need to do whatever it takes to get help quickly.

If you are using a cell phone, it becomes more difficult to track your position. **Always try to use** a regular phone to make this call. If you do reach the 911 operator with a land line, you do not need to tell the operator the address – just that you have been drugged and a man is trying to rape you. If you call from a cell phone, you will need to remain alert longer, to give a location in order to assist the police in finding you.

KNOWN ASSAILANT ATTACK SCENARIO 2:
You are at YOUR place and have just realized that **you've been drugged.** Grab a phone, then run and lock yourself inside your bathroom or bedroom. (The bedroom is better.) It is generally easier to get to one of these rooms,

rather than trying to escape, especially since you don't know what kind of drug has been administered, or how quickly you might become incapacitated. Dial 911 and **do NOT hang up** – even if the 911 operator places you on hold. Try to remain conscious. Again, throw an object through the window and scream for help by yelling, "FIRE! Please help my baby."

KNOWN ASSAILANT ATTACK SCENARIO 3: You are at his or your place and have just realized an attack is imminent **but you have not been drugged.** You absolutely need to keep your wits about you. Try to determine if you can get outside of the home or apartment before he catches you. If you don't think you can, grab a phone and run to a bedroom or bathroom and lock the door. Then dial 911. Even if the door has a working lock, place your foot at the base of the door so that it cannot be kicked open. If you cannot get a phone, throw a chair, lamp or any hard object at the nearest window to break it. DO NOT try to take the time to figure out how to open a window. Begin screaming "FIRE! Please help my baby" as loudly as you can. Neighbors will always respond to this by calling the fire department and/or the police.

Remember, 80% (4 out of 5) of all sexual assaults are committed by assailants known to the woman. In these situations where the woman knows her attacker, a strong, aggressive, boisterous response has been shown to be the most effective method to dissuade a would-be rapist. In date-rape situations, a woman should automatically default to a "getting angry" mode. This man wants to take something from you. You must make the decision that he cannot have it.

Don't forget, the *situational assailant* is not a practiced attacker. He is merely taking advantage of the situation he sees in front of him. Attacking is not really his nature as it is with the *serial assailant*. He is committing the attack based on environmental factors. If you can figure out a way to change his environment, you may very well interrupt the attack.

Example: The music is soft, the lights are low and a romantic mood has been set. He goes too far and makes it clear he plans on taking sex from you. You want to change the environment, right? So what do you do? Turn on as many lights as possible. Scream and yell at him. Push him away from you. Knock over lamps or photos. Arm yourself with any type of weapon. Do whatever it takes. These actions are now interrupting the pattern and unsettling the would-be assailant. This may also be the perfect time to quickly get out.

WEAPON SCENARIO 1: If you have access to a weapon, hold it only for *defensive* purposes. Do not try to use the weapon against your attacker. As soon as you attempt this, the weapon can be taken and used against you. Rather, hold the weapon while you are dialing 911 and tell the attacker you have just called the police. If you do not have access to a phone, use the weapon to get out of the home or apartment. **Do not turn your back on your attacker** to look for your purse. If you are in an apartment setting, get into the hallway and pull the first fire alarm lever you see. Neighbors will respond within seconds; police and firemen will respond within minutes.

WEAPON SCENARIO 2: You have access to pepper spray. Hold it out in a defensive position. Tell your attacker that you have pepper spray and you have been trained in its use. Call the police. Do not use the spray unless your attacker approaches you. You may still miss or he might block the spray; in either case you would be stuck. Use the threat of the spray as a way to guarantee your ability to move to safety or to convince your attacker that it is time for him to leave.

WEAPON SCENARIO 3: You have a gun. Do not do what they do in the movies, which is stand still while holding the gun three inches from the man's head. If someone wielding a gun is within 4 feet of someone skilled in self-defense, the gun-holder can be disarmed before ever getting the chance to fire the weapon. You must maintain a distance of at least four or five feet to ensure your safety. Grab a phone, move to a safe position such as a bedroom or bathroom or even leave the residence, then call 911.

Lately, I have been running into more and more women whose boyfriends or fathers have armed them with guns. Please understand that the use of deadly force in ANY situation carries vast repercussions. Your actions may impact you and those you care about for the rest of your lives.

If you have a gun and end up in a situation where you have decided to display it or use it, it is still best to use the weapon in a defensive manner. Say something like, "You need to leave, or I will shoot you." Say it with authority and mean it. If after making this statement, your attacker steps toward you, **you must fire the gun immediately.** His step forward is a test of whether or not you are going to allow him to take the gun from you. While maintaining the upper hand by being in possession of a gun, you should still attempt to use the few seconds where your attacker has "frozen" to grab a phone and call 911. This being said, if you are in possession of a gun or other lethal weapon, do your best to remove yourself from the situation without bringing it out into the open.

Never pull (display) a gun or any other weapon unless you are absolutely willing to use it. If an attacker takes one step toward you and you take one step back, he will know that you are not willing to use the weapon. He will attempt to take it from you. You must hold your mental and physical ground. There is nothing wrong with using a weapon to "freeze" your attacker long enough to grab a phone and run to another room or get out the door.

ABDUCTION SCENARIO 1: You have been abducted. It is essential that you do whatever you have to do to get away. **The majority of sexual abductions end in the death of the woman.** If you have been placed in a trunk, do something with the rear lights – break them, make them blink, anything to attract attention. If the car is stopped and you can hear people outside the vehicle, you must kick, scream, or do anything else you can to attract attention.

ABDUCTION SCENARIO 2: If you are driving on an open road with few populated areas and your attacker is in the car, try to blink your brake lights every time you see another vehicle approaching from the rear, especially a truck. Do this by lightly tapping on the brake pedal; not enough to slow the car, just enough to attract attention. As the car or truck passes you, look at the other driver and mouth the words "Help me!" With all the cell phones these days, someone will call the police.

ABDUCTION SCENARIO 3: If you are riding in the passenger seat of the car and your abductor has a weapon, the second the car slows down or stops, jump out and start running against the flow of traffic. Scream as loudly as you can to attract as much attention as possible. Do not look back. Get to a populated area as quickly as possible. Call the police. **IMPORTANT NOTE: Jumping out of a moving vehicle is not like on television. Even at speeds of only 5 miles per hour, jumping out of a car can result in death or serious injury.**

ABDUCTION SCENARIO 4: If you have been tied up in a trunk, your first goal is to untie yourself. Your second goal is to locate a weapon. Virtually every car has some type of jack kit (spare tire kit) located in the side walls of the trunk. Look for a screwdriver or anything else you can use. Then, when the car comes to a stop, put your body in the position you were left in, with the weapon behind your back. As soon as your abductor reaches in, stab him in the eye, chest, or groin area. You will be terrified, but you must be precise about this, because this man will kill you if you fail.

ABDUCTION SCENARIO 5: If you are driving while your abductor is in the car, get up to speed, and then slam on the brakes. Do not look to see what happens to the man, even if he has flown through the windshield. Jump out of the vehicle and run against traffic to any populated place. Call the police. If you have to crash your car into another car or a telephone pole, you need to do this. If you have to hit another car, aim for a parked car to avoid injuring an innocent person. VERY IMPORTANT: if you decide to deliberately crash your vehicle, do so at **NO MORE THAN 15 miles per hour.** The idea here is to disable the vehicle AND attract attention – NOT to injure yourself. Deliberately crashing your car will go against the grain of every part of your being, but if this attacker succeeds in removing you to a secluded location, YOU ARE GOING TO BE KILLED (almost 100% of the time).

ABDUCTION SCENARIO 6: If you are walking and a man approaches you with any kind of weapon other than a gun, run in the direction where you think the most people will be and yell "FIRE!" **If you are running from a man with a gun, instead of yelling "fire," scream "Look out. He has a gun!"** The chances of a potential abductor using the weapon as you flee is almost zero, since he knows its use will attract even more attention. He will most likely run away.

UN-ARMED ASSAILANT ATTACK SCENARIO: Your assailant is unarmed. Studies have shown that women who attempt to fight off an attacker are more likely to experience success than women who do nothing. Our natural instinct is to think, "If I cooperate, he will take what he wants and he'll leave." However, history has shown this generally not to be the case – especially with respect to sexual assaults. 84% of rape survivors tried unsuccessfully to reason with the men who raped them.[xii]

I raise this issue because studies regarding cases of sexual assaults (including interviews with incarcerated predators) have concluded that a woman's attempt to fight did not appear to make any difference to the attacker in his decision to engage in violent behavior in addition to the sexual assault itself. Meaning, in essence, that a perpetrator is no more likely to commit violence against a woman who chooses to fight back than he is against one who does not.

Therefore, the professionals have concluded: if your chances of being attacked are not increased or decreased by fighting back, you are better off attempting to physically fend off your assailant.

Other studies seem to further support this conclusion. They have shown that passive women are MORE likely to experience violent endings to a sexual assault. Rape is a crime of physical and mental domination, channeled through a sexual outlet. Pleading with an attacker, "Please don't do this" or "Please stop" only gives the attacker more of what he seeks – a sense of control and domination.

So, by all appearances, it seems that making as much noise as possible, kicking, yelling, and moving around may be more valuable than remaining passive and motionless.

Remember, if you ever find yourself in the position of being assaulted, do not yell, "Help!" or "Help me!" or other similar statements. People are understandably cautious. Even if they want to help, they have no way of knowing what they are getting themselves into, and may decide to ignore your pleas.

Screaming, "FIRE! PLEASE HELP MY BABY!" will attract people's attention every time.

In each of these scenarios, a woman's odds of thwarting an attack or preventing a completed attack increase in direct proportion to her ability to think clearly.

IN SUMMARY:

1) Do whatever you can to avoid being removed from a location by an abductor. In almost 100% of the cases, women who are abducted are subsequently killed.

2) If you have access to a weapon, use it in a defensive manner to remove yourself from a situation.

3) If you are drugged, do not think, "This will pass." Get help and get to a hospital immediately. **In a drugging situation, NEVER accept a ride from a male acquaintance** – this is most likely the person responsible for the drugging.

4) Do not yell "Help!" to attract attention; instead scream "FIRE," unless you are fleeing from an assailant with a gun.

5) Stay aware and stay sober. In the majority of cases, practicing these 2 simple habits will keep you out of harm's way.

Chapter Fifteen

The Aftermath: You Did Everything You Could, But Were Still Sexually Assaulted – What Now?

1. Remember, this was not your fault. You did not ask to be raped anymore than someone taking money out of his or her wallet asks to be robbed. **NOTHING GIVES A MAN THE RIGHT TO SEXUALLY ASSAULT A WOMAN.**

2. Report the incident **immediately,** to the police. If you are on a college campus, report it to campus security AND the police. On public school campuses, the campus police are usually duly sworn peace officers.

3. Do not wait to report. The more time that passes, the more evidence is destroyed and the less likely (I'm sorry to say) your story will be believed.

4. Do not bathe or shower.

5. Do not destroy or wash your clothing or bedding. If you remove the clothing you were wearing during the assault, place it into a paper bag – **not plastic.** Plastic bags disrupt the chemical integrity of evidence.

6. Seek medical attention as soon as possible. Your body is in shock, and you may not even be aware of an injury.

7. Seek counseling. In the immediate aftermath of a sexual assault, different women react differently. Some victims withdraw, some become depressed, some are embarrassed, others experience feelings of terror, others are resentful, and some may even blame themselves. But in virtually every incident, counseling is necessary for a woman to regain emotional balance.

8. Seriously consider following through with prosecution. Many women try to put these events behind them by making the choice not to report the crime and/or follow through with prosecution of the attacker. Understandably, many women do not want to continually "re-live" the event nor do they want to be labeled as the cause of the attack. The problem is, unless he is prosecuted, the attacker remains free to repeat the offense. I understand it is easy for me as a man to say, "Prosecute." You need to make the decision that's right for you.

See *Resources* for hotlines and counseling centers.

Thank you for reading this book. I have tried to keep it short and straightforward, while giving every woman who reads it enough information to avoid becoming another statistic.

I wish only the best for you and your loved ones.

To purchase additional copies of this book, the CD, or the © Copyrighted Scenario DVD, please visit

www.AWorldWithoutRape.org

Visit the website for special offers on all products.

Bulk discounts of books and/or CD's and/or DVD's are also available.

If you would like to have a trained professional speak to your group or institution, please contact us through the website:
www.**AWorldWithoutRape**.org

Thank you and all my best.

/s/ Richard Hart

Other books by Richard Hart

Hit the Brakes on Car Repair Rip-Offs

Award winning book showing you how to avoid rip-offs and scams, **how to minimize the likelihood of emergency situations or break-downs**, how to distinguish what is an emergency from what is not and how to recognize potential problems with your car so as to avoid being oversold or have a problem over-diagnosed.

"A must have for any person who owns or drives a car."

LifeLines: inspirational quotes on money, health, relationships and living

Book meant to inspire people to take their lives to the next level. Quotes found in this book are intended to motivate people to lead the most productive lives possible.

Perfect as an inexpensive quality gift.

You may learn more about these books or order them at:

www.**VerumPress**.com

Resources

National Sexual Assault Hotline **1 800 656 4673**.
This service is free and confidential, and available 24 hours a day, 7 days a week.

Virtually every state and county has a rape crisis hotline.

You do not need to have been the victim of a completed rape to utilize these services. Dial 411 or use an online search engine and type in the words "rape hotline your state" or "rape hotline your county."

A group called RAINN (Rape Abuse and Incest National Network). RAINN is one of the largest anti-sexual assault organizations in the country. Website: **www.RAINN.org**

You may also contact your local police department, sheriff's office or women's shelter. These entities will also have local referral numbers, websites, and support services.

Bibliography

[i]   Department of Justice as reported through the Bureau of Justice Statistics

[ii]   Bureau of Justice Statistics

[iii]   *Rape in America: A Report to the Nation*, sourced through The National Victim Center; Kilpatrick, Edmunds, and Seymour; 1992.

[iv]   Department of Justice as reported through the Bureau of Justice Statistics

[v]   United States Department of Justice; August 2000.

[vi]   *I Never Called It Rape: The Ms. Report on Recognizing, Fighting and Surviving Date and Acquaintance Rape*; Robin Warshaw; 1994; New York: Harper Perennial

[vii]   "The Mind of a Rapist," *Newsweek*; July 23, 1990.

[viii]   Warshaw

[ix]   Warshaw

[x]   Warshaw

[xi]   Department of Justice as reported through the Bureau of Justice Statistics

[xii]   Warshaw

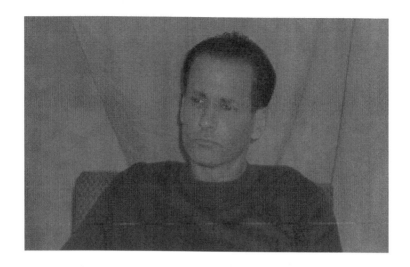

Richard Hart received a degree in Criminal Science at the age of 18. At 20 he received a B.S. from the University of California at Berkeley.

He spent five years with San Mateo Police Department and two years with Aid to Victims and Witnesses - both in a volunteer capacity. Richard was presented with an Outstanding Student Award for Community Service for these volunteer activities.

Since that time, Richard has spoken at various venues on crime prevention strategies. His unique methodology of teaching and conveying information has permitted people to avoid becoming victims of rape, robbery and other violent crimes.

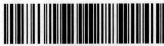

45347822R00061

Made in the USA
Lexington, KY
24 September 2015